Eat, Drink & Stay Fit:

Finding The Balance to A Healthy and Happy Life

By

Edith A. Garren

TABLE OF CONTENT

INTRODUCTION 4

CHAPTER 1 6

HOW TO SUCCESSFULLY DROP SOME WEIGHT WITHOUT HAVING TO ABANDON YOUR FAVORITE FOOD AND DRINKS 6

CHAPTER 2 19

ALCOHOL AND FAT REDUCTION 19

CHAPTER 3 29

A FITNESS PROGRAM YOU CAN DO AT HOME FOR 10 DAYS 29

HOW MUCH WEIGHT LOSS IS POSSIBLE IN TEN DAYS? 33

THE 10-DAY WORKOUT PLAN INCLUDES A VARIETY OF CARDIO EXERCISES 34

EXERCISES FOCUSING ON STRENGTH TRAINING INCLUDED IN THE 10-DAY WORKOUT PLAN 35

PROGRESSIVE LOAD: HOW TO DETERMINE WHICH WEIGHTS ARE RIGHT FOR YOU 38

WORK OUT FOR 10 DAYS 38

A SAMPLE WORKOUT PLAN FOR THE NEXT 10 DAYS 39

WHAT TO CONSUME TO LOSE TEN POUNDS IN TEN DAYS 40

ADVICE ON HOW TO MAXIMIZE THE BENEFITS OF YOUR 10-DAY WORKOUT ROUTINE 42

CHAPTER 4 44

THE PROBLEM WITH YO-YO DIETING 44

WHAT ARE THE STEPS THAT LEAD UP TO WEIGHT CYCLING? 44

THE IMPACT OF YO-YO DIETING 45

HOW TO STOP THE YO-YO EFFECT: SOME SUGGESTIONS 48

CHAPTER 5 53

WHAT SHOULD BE DONE NEXT: KEEPING A HEALTHY BODY MASS INDEX 53

HOW TO GET YOUR BMI DOWN 55

ADVANTAGES TO ONE'S HEALTH OF MAINTAINING A HEALTHY BODY MASS INDEX 57

EFFECTS OF EXERCISE ON BMI 58

PHYSICAL ACTIVITY THAT LEADS TO THE MOST SIGNIFICANT REDUCTIONS IN BMI 59

HOW TO KEEP UP A CONSISTENT PATTERN OF PHYSICAL ACTIVITY 60

OTHER ASPECTS THAT PLAY A ROLE IN DETERMINING BMI 61

THE RELATIONSHIP BETWEEN DIET AND BMI 62

IMPROVING ONE'S BODY MASS INDEX (BMI) VIA BETTER MANAGEMENT OF SLEEP AND STRESS 62

CONCLUSION 65

INTRODUCTION

The single most significant adjustment that a person can make to their diet to begin their path towards weight reduction or improve their health, in general, is to replace harmful foods with healthier ones. If you replace meals that are rich in empty calories with alternatives that are nutrient-packed yet low in calories, you will not only be able to fulfil your cravings but also aid in your weight reduction efforts. Rather than choosing quick noodles, you could select veggie noodles; peanut butter could be used in place of chocolate spread; hummus could be used in place of mayonnaise; roasted makhana could be used in place of popcorn; and butter could be used in place of margarine.

There are times when your go-to comfort meals only require a few little adjustments here and there to become healthier versions of themselves that retain the same level of flavor. Consider modifying your cooking method for various items, such as cooking meals in the oven, instead of using the traditional frying method. Switching to healthier components is another fantastic approach to improve your satisfaction from satisfying your cravings: Instead of using sugar, you may use fruit as a source of sweetness in baking a shot. To experiment successfully in the kitchen, you only need an open mind and a desire to try new things.

We all engage in behaviors, whether eating, drinking, doing things, or saying something that we know deep down isn't good for us, yet we continue to do them anyhow. Although we know these behaviors contribute to our unhappiness, we continue engaging in them as if operating on autopilot. The good news is that a prison term is not a consequence for engaging in risky behaviors. If you want to lose weight but don't want to exercise or follow a strict diet plan, there are certain things you may do, such as chewing more slowly and consuming more fiber.

CHAPTER 1

HOW TO SUCCESSFULLY DROP SOME WEIGHT WITHOUT HAVING TO ABANDON YOUR FAVORITE FOOD AND DRINKS

It might be challenging to adhere to a traditional diet and exercise regimen.

On the other hand, there are a few tried and true methods that you may use to consume fewer calories effortlessly. These are great methods for reducing your current weight and preventing you from gaining weight in the future.

All of the following fourteen methods for shedding pounds without making any changes to your eating habits or exercise routine are imperative to the objective.

Putting new, more beneficial habits that seem natural in place is the goal of habit development mechanics.

1. Chew your food thoroughly and move more slowly

It takes some time for your brain to realize that you have consumed an adequate amount of food.

You are more likely to consume the meal if you completely chew it at a slower pace, which is related to lower food intake, improved feelings of fullness, and portion control that is more appropriate for the amount of food consumed.

Your weight is also likely affected by how quickly you complete your meals.

People who did not eat very fast have a lower body mass index (BMI), as determined by a meta-analysis of the data of eight distinct pieces of study, compared to people who ate extremely quickly.

Developing the habit of eating more slowly will be easier if you keep track of the number of times throughout each meal that you chew your food.

2. Use a smaller plate whenever you are consuming foods or beverages that are high in calories.

Over the course of the last several decades, there has been a discernible increase in the size of the typical dinner plate.

Even if using a smaller plate may assist in you eating less by making servings look larger than they are, this trend could still lead to weight gain because the trend alone could trigger weight gain.

Conversely, a larger plate might make a dish appear smaller, leading you to put more food on the plate than you originally intended.

You may turn this fact to your advantage by presenting foods that are nutrient-dense but lower in calories on plates of a larger size and foods that are rich in calories on plates of a smaller size.

3. Consume a substantial amount of protein.

The consumption of protein has a significant impact on hunger. It can make you feel fuller for longer, reduce your appetite, and assist you in consuming fewer calories overall. This might be because protein affects several hormones, including ghrelin and glucagon-like peptide-1 (GLP-1), which are involved in hunger and fullness.

If you have a breakfast centered on grains, consider boosting the protein you consume at each meal.

People who consume a protein-rich breakfast, such as eggs and toast, will be less hungry later in the day and consume fewer calories overall. Compared to those who consumed a breakfast low in protein, such as cereal.

Foods such as chicken breasts, salmon, Greek yoghurt, lentils, quinoa, and almonds are a few examples of those high in protein.

4. Cook a more significant number of meals at home.

If you want to infuse more healthy foods into your diet, one of the best ways is to prepare your meals at home.

It is also possible that it will assist in the weight reduction process.

Studies have shown that people who make more of their meals at home tend to put on less weight over time than those who frequently eat out or consume prepared foods.

Meal planning may be connected with increased food quality and a lower chance of being obese.

It is recommended that you try a few different dishes each week and that you stock up on nutrient-dense items.

Making soup with broth a regular part of your diet can make you feel full while consuming fewer calories. To illustrate:

Consider minestrone, tortilla soup, or won-ton soup from China. Because it causes you to chew more slowly and reduces the amount of food you want to consume, soup is an excellent choice to start a meal with.

Boil the mixture by adding fresh or frozen veggies to a low-sodium broth or soup from a can.

Be wary of creamy soups because they may have many calories and fat.

5. Consume meals that are high in fiber.

Consuming meals high in fiber may promote satiety and help you feel fuller for a more extended period.

Viscous fiber, a specific form of roughage, may be of great assistance in the process of weight reduction. It makes you feel fuller and reduces the amount of food you eat.

When touched with water, viscous fiber transforms into a gel-like substance. This gel increases the length of time it takes for nutrients to be absorbed and decreases the rate at which your stomach empties.

Foods derived from plants are the only sources of viscous fiber. Foods such as beans, oat cereals, Brussels sprouts, asparagus, and oranges, as well as flax seeds, are foods high in fiber.

Consuming whole grains, such as brown rice, barley, oats, buckwheat, and whole wheat, should also be a component of your covert plan to lose weight. They help you feel full while consuming fewer calories and may also help reduce your cholesterol levels. Waffles, pizza crust, English muffins, spaghetti, and soft whole-wheat bread labelled "white" are some goods that now contain whole grains.

6. Make water consumption a daily habit.

It's been shown that drinking water before a meal will help you eat less overall, which can lead to weight loss.

Drinking water before a meal lessens the amount of food ingested without impacting satisfaction levels.

According to the findings of another study, drinking one pint (568 milliliters) of water before a meal will reduce the amount of calories consumed and feelings of hunger while simultaneously improving feelings of fullness and pleasure.

The impact will be amplified if you switch from consuming calorically dense beverages like soda or juice to drinking water instead.

7. Eat without being distracted by technology devices.

If you pay attention to what you put in your mouth, you could consume less calories overall.

People who consume food while viewing television or playing computer games are more likely to underestimate the quantity of food they have eaten. This, in turn, can lead to excessive food consumption.

One evaluation of 24 research published in 2013 indicated that those who were preoccupied while eating ate around 10% more food during that meal.

In addition, being distracted when eating has an even higher impact on the amount of food you consume later in the day.

You may unintentionally consume extra food if you eat meals while watching television or utilizing electronic gadgets daily. These additional calories quickly mount up and significantly influence your weight over time.

On the other hand, additional study is required because previous studies on the effects of mindful eating on food consumption have produced contradictory findings.

8. Get plenty of rest and steer clear of stress.

People frequently ignore getting enough sleep and managing their stress regarding their health. Both of these things have tremendous effects on both your hunger and your overall weight.

A disturbed balance of the hormones leptin and ghrelin, which control hunger, can be caused by a lack of sleep. When you're under pressure, your body produces more of another hormone called cortisol.

The fluctuation of these hormones can cause an increase in appetite and desire, which can lead to a greater consumption of calories.

In addition, being under constant stress and not getting enough sleep may increase your risk for several ailments, including type 2 diabetes and obesity.

According to the findings of a researcher at the University of Michigan who ran the calculations for an intake of 2,500 calories per day, sleeping an additional hour each night might assist a person in losing 14 pounds in one year. Their example demonstrates that sedentary activities, such as mindless nibbling, may be replaced with sleep, which results in a simple reduction of calorie consumption of 6%. The results would be different for each individual, but the rest might also be beneficial in another manner. Evidence suggests that having fewer than seven hours of sleep each night will stimulate your appetite, causing you to feel starving.

9. Do away with all sugary beverages.

There is an association between having a high consumption of sugar-sweetened beverages, such as fizzy drinks, and an increased risk of heart condition and type 2 diabetes.

Because drinking calories does not contribute to a feeling of fullness like eating solid food does, it is pretty simple to ingest more calories than necessary by drinking sugary beverages.

Evidence shows that reducing one's consumption of sugar-sweetened drinks can lead to weight reduction.

If you go from a sugary drink like ordinary soda to water or a sugar-free seltzer, you'll cut the sugar in your diet by roughly ten teaspoons. Try using mint, lemon, or frozen strawberries to add flavor and variety.

The liquid sugar in soda ignores the body's natural signals that it is full. One research compared an additional 450 calories daily from jelly beans to the same amount from soda. The people who ate sweets unintentionally consumed fewer calories overall, unlike those who drank soda, who consumed more. They went from losing 0.5 to gaining 2.5 pounds in that time.

According to the findings of one meta-analysis, switching from sugar-sweetened beverages to beverages with fewer calories or none at all might be associated with a reduction in BMI and ratio of body fat.

Options for beverages with fewer calories include water, unsweetened coffee or tea, and unflavored or barely sweetened green tea.

10.   Some inspirations to get you going

Hanging up your old favorite dress, skirt, or a smokin' pair of jeans in a place where you'll see them every day is a much more effective way to motivate yourself than thinking about an ex-partner, who may or may not be a motivating factor for certain individuals. This helps you retain your focus on the goal at hand.

Pick an item that fits you almost perfectly, but not quite, so you may get this prize in a reasonable amount of time. Then, dig out the cocktail dress from the previous year for your next tiny and manageable objective.

Give yourself a pat on the back when you have successfully abandoned the habit of drinking soda or just made it through the day without overeating. You are getting closer to adopting a slimming lifestyle that assists people in shedding excess weight without resorting to extreme or too complicated diet regimens. Call a friend, get a manicure, go shopping for new clothing, and treat yourself to a bite or two of cheesecake occasionally.

11. To reduce alcohol consumption and save the environment, choose tall, thin glasses and sip slowly.

If you want to reduce the number of calories you consume from liquids without having to go on a diet, try drinking from tall, narrow glasses rather than short, broad tumblers. You'll reduce your consumption of juice, soda, wine, and any other beverage by between 25 and 30 per cent.

How is this even possible? According to Brian Wansink, Ph.D., visual signals can deceive us into eating more or less. His experiments at Cornell University discovered that all types of individuals, even expert bartenders, poured more into a shorter glass that was wider at the top.

When attending an event that will involve the consumption of alcoholic beverages, it is best to follow the first drink with a nonalcoholic beverage that is low in calories, such as sparkling water, rather than going straight to another cocktail, beer, or glass of wine. There are seven times as many calories in one gram of alcohol than there are in carbs (4) or protein (4). Additionally, it might weaken your determination, which can cause you to mindlessly devour meals like chips, almonds, and other items you would ordinarily limit.

Consuming green tea may also be beneficial for weight loss. According to certain research findings, it can temporarily rev up the body's calorie-burning engine, presumably due to the activity of phytochemicals known as catechins. You will, at the absolute least, receive a beverage that is cooling and does not contain a large number of calories.

12.   The particular rule of 80/20

In the United States, people are socialized to keep eating until they are filled up; however, in Okinawa, they stop eating when they are just 80% satisfied. They even have a term for this natural weight loss practice, and it's called hara hachi bu. We may implement This healthy practice by reducing the food we serve by 20%.

13.   Allow Yourself One Cheat Meal Consisting of Your Favorite Food

Every weight-loss regimen requires a "cheat meal" once a week. If you are following a diet plan that requires you to permanently abstain from eating one of your favorite foods, then you are most likely doing so incorrectly. Cheat meals are critical for resetting your metabolism, satisfying cravings, preventing binge eating, breaking through weight loss plateaus, and, most significantly, improving your ability to adhere to your diet plan more effectively. It is a reward-based diet plan that allows you to indulge in your preferred cuisine outside of your diet program once a week and also paves the way for the burning of additional excess body fat in the long run. Because of this, the Rati Beauty plan recommends allowing yourself one cheat meal every week so that you may continue to make progress toward your weight reduction goals. Do you desire more than one taste of those glazed doughnuts, or would you like to consume pizza? Consume these in place of your regular meal!

14. Be sure to get up and move about and exercise daily.

The advantages of physical activity on one's health are numerous and varied, ranging from reducing stress and enhancing memory to facilitating improved sleep quality. The main benefit, however, in terms of managing your weight is the acceleration of the calories that are burned by your body. When you are hankering for one of your favorite foods but know that you are burning a few additional calories, you may indulge in that cuisine without feeling guilty. It would be best if you were consistent with the physical exercise you choose. In addition to assisting with weight loss, physical activity has been shown to boost overall satisfaction and foster the mentality necessary to adopt healthy eating habits.

KEY POINT

It's feasible to maintain your current eating habits while still attaining your weight loss objectives; the key is to strike a healthy balance. The adage "everything in moderation" may be dull, but it's sound advice that may be put to good use. You can cultivate a more positive and long-term healthy relationship with food if you can have your cake and eat it, also, provided that you do it consciously, slowly, and in moderation. If you choose to follow restrictive diets and cut out all of your favorite foods, you will end up gaining the weight back until you reach the point when you can no longer resist things like cake.

There are several straightforward modifications to one's lifestyle that might facilitate weight loss. Some of these strategies have nothing to do with the traditional approaches to dieting or working out.

Eating off smaller plates, taking your time, drinking extra water, and steering clear of eating in front of the television or computer. Putting meals high in protein and viscous fiber at the forefront of your diet may also be helpful.

On the other hand, it probably would be better to test out all of these things at different times. Experiment with one method for a while to see how well it works for you; if that method succeeds, go on to the next.

A few uncomplicated adjustments influence your weight over time.

Following all the earlier outlined points will assist you tremendously.

CHAPTER 2

ALCOHOL AND FAT REDUCTION

Although the connection between drinking alcohol and being overweight has not been definitively established, there is compelling evidence to suggest that alcohol may have a role in both conditions.

- It prevents your body from burning the fat that it already has. It has a high kilojoule content.
- It causes an increase in appetite and a decrease in satiety (feeling of being full).
- It can cause an urge to eat salty and oily foods.

Because alcohol frequently includes "empty calories" and can affect your organ systems, cutting back on how much of it you drink could make it easier to lose weight.

The alcohol is processed by your body much like a toxin. For your body to concentrate on metabolizing the alcohol, it shuts down all of your other metabolic pathways. Depending on the amount consumed and the person, drinking alcohol might inhibit the body's ability to burn fat for anywhere between 12 and 36 hours. People are advised to limit their drinking to the day before and the day of their cheat day. Since you are not trying to reduce body fat on your cheat day, drinking alcohol on such nights will not slow your progress toward your goals. Consuming alcohol on days not designated as cheat days can slow the rate at which you lose weight. Adjust your expectations for weight reduction and take responsibility if you consume alcohol on days not designated as cheat days.

Your liver may have an easier time metabolizing alcohol if you follow a diet low in carbohydrates, as much as two to three times more effective.

Consuming alcoholic beverages is a common human pastime that is highly valued in both social and cultural contexts.

Others maintain that drinking alcohol can be beneficial to one's health. For instance, drinking red wine may reduce the likelihood of getting heart disease.

However, alcohol consumption also significantly impacts the control of one's weight. If you're trying to eliminate those last few pounds that won't disappear, missing that glass of wine with dinner could be the best option.

Here are eight ways that drinking alcohol might get in the way of your efforts to lose weight, along with some suggestions for alternatives.

1. Many times, the calories from alcohol are "empty" calories

Many people consider the calories in alcoholic beverages to be "empty" calories. This indicates that they are a source of calories for your body but offer relatively few other nutritional benefits.

Alcohol has seven calories per gram, roughly twice as much as the four calories in protein and three in carbs. There are only two fewer calories in alcohol per gram than in fat, which comprises nine calories. It is crucial to keep in mind that alcohol does not include any of the nutrients that are necessary for a healthy metabolism, and as a result, drinking alcohol will speed up the process of fat storage.

Because of the high concentration of calories that may be found in the typical alcoholic beverage compared to the calories present in many meals, drinking alcohol can induce a person to unintentionally ingest a great deal more calories than they usually would. Alcohol is quite misleading because it moves through the system quickly, so the person drinking it is frequently unaware of how many drinks they already have.

A single can of beer that is 12 ounces contains about 155 calories, whereas a glass of red wine that is 5 ounces contains 125 calories. In perspective, the ideal calorie count for an afternoon snack is between 150 and 200. A night out with numerous drinks might increase several hundred calories in one's daily calorie intake.

Drinks with mixers, such as fizzy drinks, have an even higher calorie content than those consumed independently.

2. A fundamental source of energy, alcohol is employed in the production of fuel

In addition to the number of calories something contains, additional factors can play a role in weight growth.

When alcohol is taken into the body, it is metabolized as fuel before anything else is used. This contains glucose, which is derived from carbs, as well as lipids, which are derived from fats.

The extra glucose and lipids that are produced when your body uses alcohol as its primary source of energy are stored, sadly for us, as adipose tissue, which is another name for fat.

3. Consuming alcohol might have an impact on your organs

Your liver's principal function is to "filter" any foreign chemicals, such as drugs and alcohol, that make their way into your system. This includes any toxins. Additionally, the liver is involved in the body's breakdown of carbohydrates, proteins, and lipids.

Consuming excessive alcohol might result in a condition known as alcoholic fatty liver.

This disorder can cause damage to your liver, which can impact how your body metabolizes carbs and lipids as well as how it stores them.

Alterations in how the body stores energy obtained from eating might make it exceedingly challenging to lose weight.

4. Consuming alcohol can lead to having a larger than the regular waistline

The so-called "beer gut" is more than just an urban legend.

The number of calories in foods heavy in simple sugars, such as candy, soda, and beer, is likewise high. Extra calories are transformed into fat and stored throughout the body.

A rapid increase in weight gain is possible when one consumes meals and drinks heavy in sugar.

We do not get a say in the matter of where all of that extra weight goes. On the other hand, the human body tends to store fat in the abdominal region.

5. Consuming alcohol impairs one's judgment, particularly regarding eating

When under the influence of alcohol, it will be difficult for anyone, no matter how dedicated they are to their diet, to resist the impulse to dive in.

Consuming alcohol reduces one's inhibitions, which can result in bad decisions in the heat of the moment, particularly concerning one's selection of foods.

Because drinking alcohol can stimulate hunger, combining it with a meal high in calories can have an even more detrimental effect. Drinking alcohol before a meal will lead to a far more significant increase in calories taken than sipping a beverage containing carbohydrates.

6. Sexual hormones and alcoholic beverages

It has been known for a very long time that drinking alcohol can alter the quantities of hormones found in the body, particularly testosterone.

Testosterone is a sex hormone involved in various metabolic activities, including the ability to build muscle and burn fat.

Consuming alcohol causes a reduction in testosterone, which has a profound influence on fat loss. Because of this, testosterone cannot reach its full potential as a fat burner. Testosterone's anabolic properties also contribute to increases in total and lean muscle mass. A reduction in levels of testosterone leads to a decrease in muscle growth, and a reduction in muscle leads to a slowing metabolic rate.

A slower metabolic rate will make shedding fat much more challenging to accomplish. This is what determines how we consume energy in our society. Those who have a greater metabolic rate will burn more calories when their body is at rest. Alcohol indirectly causes a decrease in the body's metabolic rate (and, as a result, the pace at which it utilizes energy), and alcohol directly prevents testosterone from exerting the tremendous fat-burning effects that it is capable of. Alcohol does this by interfering with the creation of testosterone.

Based on their low testosterone levels, it is possible to anticipate the presence of metabolic syndrome in males. The following factors contribute to the development of metabolic syndrome:

High cholesterol levels

High blood pressure

High blood sugar levels

A high body mass index

In addition, having reduced amounts of testosterone may impact sleep quality, particularly in older men.

7. Consuming alcohol might have a detrimental impact on the quality of your sleep

You might think that having one last drink before bed would help you get a good night's sleep, but you should rethink that decision.

Drinking alcohol can result in more prolonged spells of awake during a regular night's sleep.

A disparity in the hormones that regulate appetite, fullness, and energy storage can result from not getting enough sleep, whether that sleep loss is caused by not sleeping or being unable to sleep.

8. Consuming alcohol disrupts digestion and the absorption of nutrients

Inhibiting your social anxiety is only one of the many things alcohol does. Consuming alcoholic drinks might also hinder digestion if done in excess.

Consuming alcohol can put a strain on both the digestive tract and the stomach. This reduces the amount of digestive fluids produced and slows down the transit of food through the digestive system.

The digestive tract cannot function properly without the secretions the digestive organs produce. They disassemble the meal into its component macro- and micronutrients, which are then absorbed by the body and used by it.

Any amount of alcohol use might result in a reduction in the body's ability to digest and absorb these nutrients. This can have a significant impact on the metabolic processes of organs that are involved in the regulation of body weight.

The most effective alcoholic beverages for weight reduction

All of this may make it seem like drinking alcohol destroys your chances of having a beach body. However, you shouldn't panic since if you want to control your weight, it doesn't always imply that you have to eliminate alcohol from your diet.

Instead of reaching for beverages that are rich in sugar or calories, try some of these other alternatives that are just 100 calories each:

- There are 100 calories in 1.5 ounces of distilled 80-proof vodka. Alternative cocktail: Choose mixers with fewer calories, such as club soda, and steer clear of juices with excessive sugar.
- The amount of calories in whisky is as follows: 100 calories in 1.5 ounces of an 86-proof whisky option cocktail. Consume your whisky on the rocks rather than with cola for a low-calorie option.
- The equivalent of one and a half ounces of 90-proof gin contains 115 calories. An alternative drink would be A straightforward option such as a martini is recommended; nevertheless, you shouldn't leave out the olives because they are packed with healthy antioxidants like vitamin E.
- The average "shot" of tequila consists of simply salt, tequila, and lime juice. This is one of the most excellent things about

tequila since it only has 100 calories per 1.5 ounces of alcohol.

Alternative cocktail: This drink is ideally served as an after-dinner digestif, and a fine brandy should be drunk slowly to savor the nuanced fruity sweetness it contains. There are about 100 calories in 1.5 ounces of brandy.

KEY POINT

Is it possible to abstain from the use of alcohol, given the significant role it plays in the process of celebrating and maintaining social cohesion? It highly depends on the objectives a person has set for themselves. Most people generally wouldn't experience any adverse effects from drinking alcohol in modest amounts (two or three standard drinks three to four times per week).

While eliminating alcohol from your diet entirely isn't necessarily the only method to lose weight, merely cutting back on your use of alcoholic beverages can lead to significant benefits in your overall health and wellness journey.

A healthier body, greater sleep, enhanced digestion, and reduced "empty" calories you consume in excess are all possible benefits.

And if you are going to drink, we recommend having a whisky or vodka on the rocks rather than a soda.

Also, you should try to be consistent with your cheat days even with your alcohol intake.

Try as much as possible to resist the urge of deviating from your routine and find alternatives.

CHAPTER 3

A FITNESS PROGRAM YOU CAN DO AT HOME FOR 10 DAYS

The topic of losing weight is important to a lot of individuals. It may seem intimidating, challenging, and time-consuming, but if you are determined and have the time and energy to spend, learning how to get in shape in as little as two weeks is achievable.

Find a workout routine that works for you, make good food choices, and consume a lot of water, and then see how your body starts to change.

Do you find yourself fascinated by famous people? Who are these flawless individuals who can shed their baby weight in a couple of weeks and then flaunt their toned stomachs while lounging on a beach in Ibiza? We put ourselves through unnecessary stress by striving to replicate the same unachievable performance. Actors can reach their physical objectives more quickly when they follow the tried-and-true formula of keeping a great diet, participating in regular exercise, and getting adequate rest, mainly when a team of trained professionals backs them. "The importance of nutrition will increase the closer you reach your objective.

Modifying your lifestyle and making a few changes are the solutions to successful weight loss and improved physical fitness. Following these simple weight loss techniques, you may lose between 2 and 3 kilograms in ten days.

Take in some water.

Drink plenty of water throughout the day to keep yourself hydrated. Water plays a significant part in helping the body wash out harmful pollutants.

The first thing you should do when you get up is drink water. This will start your metabolism going. It is also helpful in controlling the hunger sensations that lead to an insatiable need for food.

After eating, go for a walk.

After eating, a little stroll for just five minutes assists digestion and contributes to losing some calories. It has been shown that going for a walk after eating can assist in the removal of glucose from the bloodstream to some degree. This is because the muscles consume a significant portion of it to carry out their duties.

Eat extra fiber, and reduce added sugars.

Complex carbs, such as those found in whole grains, legumes, fruits, and vegetables; healthy fats, like those found in nuts, seeds, and avocados; and plenty of lean proteins, low in saturated and trans fats (bring on the chicken and fish!). These are the diet's main components most suited to sustain an intensive exercise schedule.

Eat more veggies, salads, and soups to improve your health. One of your meals should consist solely of veggies or sprouts. Reduce your consumption of cereals after 7 o'clock. Munch on some fruits, seeds, nuts, or chana for a snack. Also, steer clear of alcoholic beverages as much as is humanly feasible.

Perform a calorie count

The number of calories consumed on a diet should be adjusted according to the goals of the diet. If someone wants to put on muscle, they need to finish more than they burn off, but if they're going to lose weight, they need to eat fewer calories.

Observe the macros

Maintaining track of carbohydrate, fat, and protein macros is crucial, especially considering protein is the most significant nutrient for increasing muscle mass. However, many dietitians and bodybuilders advocate raising that up to 0.8 to 1 gram for people aiming to grow and retain muscle. The recommended daily requirement for protein is between 0.31 and 0.45 grams per pound of body weight.

In-house dining

This is a no-brainer of a decision. Our more experienced peers have instructed us to eat food prepared at home.

People commonly eat their meals away from home or prepare food to eat later because of the hectic lifestyles that people lead today. On the other hand, these kinds of foods are frequently quite heavy in fat and oil, and as a result, eating them regularly might cause you to gain weight unhealthfully over time. When you cook at home, you have complete control over what goes into your dish, unlike when you eat out.

Eat less salty foods

It would be best to stock up on only some processed goods sold over the counter. This contains snacks such as chips, cookies, and other similar foods. These include a great amount of salt, which is added so they will stay good quickly. Consuming excessive salt might cause you to appear and feel bloated.

Exercise: Make it a daily habit to participate in physical activity for at least half an hour. This is one of the finest ways to reduce weight without causing any harm to the body, especially when combined with a balanced diet. Choose a workout regimen that suits your time constraints and preferences. The best results may be achieved by combining resistance training with cardiovascular exercise. When the goal is to seem stronger in a short amount of time, the workouts typically concentrate more on weightlifting. If you want to appear leaner rather than bulkier or have more time to devote to your workouts, the exercise plan might involve more cardiovascular activity.

Get some rest

Because food and exercise may be affected by sleep, anyone aiming to get in shape quickly should shoot for at least seven hours of sleep every night. Not only does a lack of sleep contribute to overeating due to sleep's influence on the neurotransmitters that tell when it's time to stop eating, but a lack of sleep also prevents muscular regeneration and saps one's energy levels. On the other hand, getting adequate sleep helps control eating, promotes muscular building, and offers the energy to visit the gym once again.

If you keep up with this routine, you should notice benefits within a few days at the latest.

HOW MUCH WEIGHT LOSS IS POSSIBLE IN TEN DAYS?

Everyone will give you a different response if you ask them this question. Your weight may shift depending on the intensity of your exercises, the quantity of food you consume, and the phase of the moon. Several factors, including the following, influence your ability to lose weight:

- Your current health status
- The weight that you want to achieve
- Height/weight ratio = BMI (body mass index);
- Sex-related characteristics such as pregnancy or menopause.
- Rate of metabolism
- Activity level
- Age
- Height/weight ratio = BMI (body mass index).

You need to determine how much weight you want to lose, your ideal weight, and how long it will take you to get there before you can analyze your weight reduction objectives. An excellent goal for some individuals may be to lose five to ten pounds in ten days. For the rest, 14-21 pounds would be more appropriate.

Depending on the specifics of the individual's situation, as stated above, a healthy rate of weight reduction would be anything from half a pound to two pounds lost every week.

THE 10-DAY WORKOUT PLAN INCLUDES A VARIETY OF CARDIO EXERCISES

One of the finest things you can do for your body is engage in daily physical activity. Workouts that focus on aerobic movement, often known as cardio, are beneficial for many reasons outside of weight reduction, including the following:

- Decreased levels of stress
- Lower blood pressure and cholesterol levels, which lower the risk of heart disease
- Improved bone density and posture
- Increased levels of energy
- Improved mental concentration

Because doing cardio raises your metabolic rate, you will continually burn calories even after you finish your workout for the rest of the day if you do it regularly. If you are searching for a fitness regimen that can help you lose weight in ten days, you might consider including some jogging in the routine. Keep it brief: running for little more than

half an hour twice a week is all that is necessary to see positive outcomes.

The following great cardio activities should be included in your workout routine: treadmill workouts, mountain climbers, jumping jacks, burpees, and shadow boxing.

Your cardiovascular activity should begin with a warm-up that lasts ten minutes. This will increase the pace at which your heart beats and cause you to burn additional calories, allowing you to maximize your progress for the following thirty minutes. After your last cooling exercise session of another ten minutes, which should be stretching, you should finish by gradually lowering your heart rate.

EXERCISES FOCUSING ON STRENGTH TRAINING INCLUDED IN THE 10-DAY WORKOUT PLAN

Workouts that focus on building lean muscle mass are ideal for weight loss because they increase the body's metabolic rate, allowing for more calories to be burnt even though the body is sitting for most of the day.

Research has indicated that moderate strength training can increase one's overall sense of well-being by triggering the release of endorphins throughout the body. This might be beneficial if you feel like you need a little additional motivation to start your weight loss journey.

Strength training is advantageous for some reasons; one is that it helps improve muscular strength, which builds up muscles and bones, reducing the risk of injury.

Concentrating on fundamental exercises like squats, deadlifts, rows, presses, and pull-ups/chin-ups is the most effective strategy for developing a regimen for strength training.

When performed with the correct technique, these exercises have been shown, for decades of research in various settings with people from novices to athletes, men and women alike, to be effective at growing muscle growth while reducing injury.

You should strive to complete three sets of eight repetitions with a minute of rest between each set. This will ensure your weights are doable while providing sufficient time to build up your endurance for each exercise.

Some of the most effective workouts for developing muscular strength include:

Lunges

You may perform these workouts at home or in a fitness center. You don't need to leave your house for a good lunge workout; you only need some dumbbells. Taking dumbbells in both hands, step forward into a lunge stance and then return to a standing position to complete the exercise.

Squats

Because you are utilizing all of the muscles in your lower body to stabilize yourself as you lower yourself from an upright posture, simple squats can help you tone muscles across your entire body. This workout may be made more difficult by adding weight, holding dumbbells, or wearing a rucksack with weights. If you want more of a challenge, consider adding weight.

Deadlifts

The glutes, legs, core, arms, and back muscles, to mention a few, are among the many muscle groups that benefit from performing deadlifts since they require lifting heavy things. You will only need a barbell and some weights to get started.

Row

You'll get the best possible results from rowing exercises if you use dumbbells, but if you don't have access to dumbbells, you may substitute resistance bands for the dumbbells instead. Your triceps, your lats, and your forearms will all get a workout with this upper-body exercise. You can perform the activity while seated or standing, depending on the variation you are attempting to accomplish.

Press

This exercise requires you to push a weight away from yourself during any press performed for this workout, whether sitting or standing. Presses engage various muscles, including the triceps, shoulders, pecs, abdominals, and legs. If increasing your muscle mass is one of your goals, you should be sure not to skip presses since more lean muscle results in a faster metabolic rate. In addition, it means acquiring greater strength and coordination, which are beneficial in reducing the risk of injury while engaging in regular physical activity.

Perform pull-ups and chin-ups.

The rhomboids, lats, and trapezius muscles in your back will all get a workout from these workouts. You may perform pull-ups or chin-ups using a straight bar that is weighted if feasible to make it more challenging. Therefore, try out both types and push yourself as far as you need to be pushed while taking care not to harm yourself.

Extensions of the back

While performing this exercise, you may work on strengthening your core and lower back by elevating your legs, chest, and upper body off the ground. Because this is an advanced form of the workout, you should begin by performing abdominal crunches before adding weight as a weight belt or a weighted backpack.

PROGRESSIVE LOAD: HOW TO DETERMINE WHICH WEIGHTS ARE RIGHT FOR YOU

To determine how much weight you should lift for your chosen activity, begin with the least weight feasible and make it a goal to gradually increase it as you go through each of your workouts. Find personal trainers in your region who focus on strength training if you need assistance calculating how much weight you should be lifting. Alternatively, ask a reliable friend or member of your family to spot you while you work out so that you don't injure yourself.

WORK OUT FOR 10 DAYS

You should make the following your priority for the next ten days:

1-2 Sessions of Cardio Workouts

When you aim to lose 10 pounds in 10 days, keep your cardio sessions as brief and strenuous as possible.

As an illustration, set a goal of running for a combined period of thirty minutes. If you are not a runner, you should choose another kind of cardiovascular exercise that is difficult but within your capabilities, such as swimming or biking. Cycling is a fantastic exercise since, unlike running, it does not stress the joints.

Strength Training: 3 sets of 8 reps with a 60-second rest period between each set

If you want to grow muscle while minimizing the risk of injury during your workouts, you should ensure that your routine includes the exercises described. Your strength training regimen can also include high-intensity interval training (HIIT), which has been demonstrated to enhance metabolic rate and burn fat once a workout is over. HIIT stands for high-intensity interval training. Those pressed for time will find that HIIT is an excellent option.

A SAMPLE WORKOUT PLAN FOR THE NEXT 10 DAYS
The following is an example of a 10-day workout schedule that you may use:

- On Monday, you'll focus on upper and lower-body pull exercises (such as chest presses, lateral lifts, and overhead presses).

- Upper body pulls and lower body pushes on Tuesday (such as dumbbell pullovers, bicep curls, pull-ups, and squats, for example).
- Wednesday is a day of rest.
- Upper body push followed by lower body pull on Thursday (chest flies, single leg deadlifts, dumbbell snatches).
- On Friday, you'll work your upper body with pulling exercises and your lower body with pushing exercises (barbell curls, single arm rows, raised step-ups).
- On Saturdays, we do cardio using LISS.
- Cardio HIIT over the weekend
- On Monday, you will focus on upper-body push exercises and lower-body pull exercises, such as chest flies, single-leg deadlifts, and dumbbell snatches.
- On Tuesday, you'll work your upper body with pulling exercises and your lower body with pushing exercises (barbell curls, single arm rows, raised step-ups).
- Wednesday is a day of rest.

WHAT TO CONSUME TO LOSE TEN POUNDS IN TEN DAYS

Diet and exercise are both important factors in successful weight loss. This is the food that you ought to consume:

Protein Devoid of Excess Fat

When attempting to lose weight for ten days, you must consume a lot of protein so your body has enough components necessary for creating muscle.

Because it reduces abdominal fat, consuming a protein-rich diet will also help reduce inflammation and the likelihood of developing insulin resistance, lowering the risk of other chronic diseases.

Vegetables High in Fiber

Your goal should be to consume as many green veggies as possible because they are low in calories but high in nutrients. This indicates that they contain a significant quantity of nutrients concerning their caloric value, which is determined by the thermic effect of food, also known as TEF.

Carbohydrates of a Complicated Nature

Carbohydrates have had a bad rap in recent years, but certain carbohydrates are superior to others. Your goal should be to steer clear of refined carbohydrates like refined sugar and white and instead go with carbohydrates from fruits and whole grains.

Fats

Some fats are required for proper brain function and for maintaining the health of the nervous system, while others, such as trans fats, should be avoided at all costs. Each kind of fat plays a unique and vital role in the body. Nuts, seeds, avocados, butter from grass-fed cows, olive oil, and other healthy fats may be found in foods like these.

The water

As discussed earlier, you should make it a point to consume sufficient water daily since this is one of the most important things you can do for your overall health and wellness.

ADVICE ON HOW TO MAXIMIZE THE BENEFITS OF YOUR 10-DAY WORKOUT ROUTINE

Consume a Great Deal of Protein

Aim to achieve 0.8 grams of protein for every pound of lean mass, which equals 154 grams for every 75 kilograms. This will guarantee that your muscles can repair themselves before your workout, maximizing your muscular growth.

Take some days off

Because your muscles require building time, you should avoid exercising daily for the first ten days. If you continue to do that, your strength will gradually decrease, so make sure you give yourself at least one to two days of relaxation per week.

Consume Dietary Supplements

Consuming the appropriate supplements can assist in maximizing muscle growth, energy levels, and recuperation times. Amino acids are needed for the mixture of protein, whereas branched-chain amino acids, often known as BCAAs, are necessary for restoring the pH balance of the blood after severe workouts, the kind that might make you want to stop exercising prematurely. Before, during, and after physical activity, maintaining a healthy vitamin balance in the body is essential for optimal health and well-being. Taking a high-quality multivitamin supplement can help you do just that.

Sleep

The ability of your cells to renew and proliferate in response to the demands of high-intensity training is directly correlated to the amount of sleep you get each night. Sleep deficiency leads to a reduction in the synthesis of growth hormone and testosterone in the body, resulting in a retardation of muscle development. When trying to lose weight in a week, you should shoot for between 7 and 9 hours of sleep each night.

KEY POINT

If you stick to a balanced diet and an exercise routine, you may lose anywhere from five to ten pounds of fat in ten days. Combination strength training with high-intensity interval training (HIIT) is the most effective methodology to accomplish this goal since it promotes the greatest amount of muscle building while simultaneously reducing body fat. A fantastic place to get started is with the 10-day fitness challenge.

CHAPTER 4

THE PROBLEM WITH YO-YO DIETING

The so-called yo-yo effect is a challenging obstacle many individuals must overcome when attempting to reduce weight.

The clinical word for yo-yo dieting is "weight cycling," which implies inadvertently gaining weight, dieting as a response to that weight gain, and then regaining that weight again. Yo-yo dieting is also referred to as "weight cycling." After that, you start another attempt at losing weight by dieting, and the process continues.

This never-ending cycle of dieting is brought on by the constant social pressure to maintain a healthy weight in a society obsessed with diets. Although we are prone to regaining the weight we lose, many of us succumb to the delusion that the next diet will be different or that, this time, we will have more resolve to keep the weight off permanently. But is it the case that you need a new strategy or just need to be more disciplined?

WHAT ARE THE STEPS THAT LEAD UP TO WEIGHT CYCLING?

The pressure and the desire to be smaller can be the impetus for yo-yo dieting, which leads to a never-ending struggle to fight against our biology. Because of this, there will undoubtedly be consistent shifts in our weight over time. And this makes perfect sense, considering that we live in a culture that places an extremely high value on being skinny.

Results from crash diets are frequently temporary and not sustainable. The primary types of lost weight are water weight and muscle mass. Following this, your metabolic rate will decrease due to restricting calories and losing muscle mass.

After going on a diet, if you immediately return to your former eating and lifestyle habits, you will quickly put the weight you lost back on since your basal metabolic rate (BMR) has decreased due to eating fewer calories. After that, your body will store the calories it receives from food as fat. Therefore, the mechanism that underlies the yo-yo effect is an essential defensive function that shields the body from bouts of hunger.

Your body weight may even wind up being much higher than it was before you started the diet. This is because the quantity of muscle mass you lose, your BMR, and how soon you go back to your former eating habits are all factors that influence your body weight.

THE IMPACT OF YO-YO DIETING
Reduced rate of metabolism

Your body truly perceives the diet you are following as a "famine," which may surprise you. Because natural selection has allowed the body to quickly learn how to tolerate states of 'famine,' the body is unable to differentiate between actual starving and starvation, which is self-inflicted and down-regulating non-essential activities such as bone metabolism, reproductive function, and the preservation of hair or nails. After the so-called "fasting" period has ended, the body will make an effort to restore its metabolism to its pre-"fasting" level. However, the body's success in doing so will be hindered by the loss of lean muscle tissue that occurred during the weight loss phase (we will discuss this further in a moment). During the phase of weight return, we observe that fat is gained much more quickly than muscle mass, with an increased quantity of fat distributed as visceral fat, which surrounds essential organs within the belly. Additionally, the body has an increase in the total amount of fat overall. This preferred fat storage can be considered a survival mechanism to store more energy away in preparation for the next period when food is lacking.

wasting away the muscle's lean mass

When you go on a diet, your body will burn the fat reserved in your body for fuel and destroy the lean muscle tissue you have if it is not obtaining enough energy. This is due to the fact that your central nervous system, red blood cells, etc., can only operate well if they are given glucose to consume as a source of fuel. Because they cannot store glucose as our muscles and other organs do, they require a consistent supply of glucose from our meals. If there is not enough glucose in the body, the body will adjust by engaging in a process known as gluconeogenesis, which involves converting amino acids taken from the muscle tissue into glucose. Your metabolic rate will decline even further if you lose any more lean muscle tissue.

Increased levels of the stress hormone hydrocortisone in our bodies

A diet, sometimes known as semi-starvation, may be a stressful experience for our bodies. Elevated cortisol levels can bring on a greater capacity for fat accumulation and an increase in hunger. This makes perfect sense when viewed through the lens of evolutionary theory. When we are under a lot of pressure, our bodies mistakenly believe we are in imminent danger. As a result, they begin to stockpile fat in preparation for the possibility that we would require more energy to fend off an attacker. In the past, this danger may have been posed by a tiger or a hostile tribe. However, in the advanced society that we live in today, the dangers we face are entirely different, and they frequently manifest themselves in the shape of ongoing duties such as job, school, and family obligations.

Techniques for losing weight that are not healthy.

Inappropriate strategies for weight loss, such as a lack of suitable exercise and the use of weight loss drugs, eventually result in greater risks of having the yo-yo dieting pattern. It is possible that the yo-yo effect will not typically be evident during the initial weight control program, particularly in young, healthy individuals. However, if these unhealthy weight loss behaviors are sustained, losing weight becomes progressively more difficult, frequently resulting in a cycle of weight gain and loss known as the yo-yo effect.

Diets that involve cutting calories or skipping meals

Although cutting calorie consumption fast leads to weight loss, this is attributable to a decrease in muscle mass rather than body fat. When you lose muscle mass, your body will naturally adjust by slowing your metabolism to compensate for the change. Experts believe that a slower metabolism may be a factor in why people lose weight after abandoning low-calorie diets and eating normally again. As metabolic function declines, it becomes more difficult to lose weight. This is because of the weight loss plateau.

HOW TO STOP THE YO-YO EFFECT: SOME SUGGESTIONS

If you have your heart set on shedding some pounds, this up-and-down cycle might make you feel like a complete and utter failure.

However, there is an exit from the roller coaster. Improving one's health and happiness is feasible by avoiding the latest trends, putting in the necessary mental effort, and coming out on top. Stop beating yourself up and telling yourself you're a loser because you couldn't follow a crazy new diet plan.

The first steps are as follows.

1. Stay away from crash diets.

Put low-carb diets and other trendy eating plans out of your mind! Extreme diets that cut out whole food categories or drastically restrict the amount of calories consumed will not provide long-lasting benefits. What takes place? You revert to your previous habits and experience rapid weight gain.

To lose weight healthily and sustainably, you might consider a moderate calorie reduction (between 300 and 500 calories per day). It is reasonable to aim to lose roughly half a kilogram every week, and doing so will aid you in keeping your weight low.

2. Guard your balance and ensure that you get enough to eat

You must eat enough food to lose weight and keep it off long-term. If you make long-term changes to your diet and eat in an instinctively balanced way, you will significantly improve your chances of avoiding the yo-yo effect. Listening to your body is an integral part of eating intuitively. There are no restricted foods; one may eat whatever they want without feeling bad.

Consuming adequate fiber, protein, and high-quality fats can replenish your body and relieve cravings.

3. Boost your standard basal metabolic rate

Your BMR is the energy your body requires to carry out all of its necessary processes. It will fall if you don't consume enough calories during the day. Because your metabolism enters a state of famine, you won't be able to shed any pounds. What options do you have? Building muscle mass will increase your BMR. While you move, your muscles burn glucose and fat; this process continues even while you sleep. Building and keeping a suitable amount of muscle mass is the only method to cut calories and prevent the yo-yo effect from occurring when dieting.

4. Keep moving during the day

Increasing the calories you burn during the day may be accomplished by including regular exercise. Take your bike instead of your car more often, go for regular walks, avoid using lifts and escalators in favor of the stairs, and leave your car at home more regularly. This is something that is not only beneficial to your physical health but also wonderful for your spirit. In addition, being outside in the fresh air and sunshine helps your immune system, and getting adequate amounts of vitamin D is needed for good health.

5. Ensure that you get plenty of rest

Your likelihood of being obese and gaining weight increases if you do not get enough sleep and have a high-stress level. The yo-yo effect may be avoided effectively following weight reduction by taking steps to reduce stress. Exercising can lower stress levels. Remember that adults require between seven and nine hours of sleep every night to maintain good health.

6. Seek help

Utilize the knowledge of an individual knowledgeable in the subject matter and can advise you along the path, whether your objective is to reduce your weight or to adopt better habits that will enhance your health (with or without weight reduction as the final aim). There is an impression that you can handle things on your own. Stop being so hard on yourself. It is not at all inappropriate to look for assistance.

In conclusion, to prevent the yo-yo effect, the following suggestions for a healthy weight reduction program should be followed:

- Decrease overall body fat while maintaining muscle mass
- It is imperative that you do not skip meals, reduce the amount of food you consume, and increase the proportion of low-calorie items in your diet.
- Stay away from diets that are heavy in calories and fat, such as meals that are fried in oil, whether they are deep-fried or pan-fried.
- Maintain a regular exercise routine and make appropriate dietary adjustments. You should get at least 150 minutes of activity each week, especially during the first six months of your pregnancy. To keep a healthy weight while engaging in long-term weight management, the amount of time spent exercising should be raised to between 200 and 300 minutes per week, and this increase should be maintained consistently for at least a year.
- Begin using nutritional self-monitoring tools, such as a journal of daily foods and weight reduction trends, to increase your chances of successfully controlling your weight over the long run.
- It is strongly encouraged to consult with nutritionists and dieticians at least once monthly to guarantee that healthy weight management programs are appropriately

implemented for sustained weight reduction without harming general health.

KEY POINT

Changing some of our more ingrained eating habits may be tricky, making weight reduction difficult. However, to successfully and permanently reduce weight, it is necessary to employ promising approaches for weight reduction. The importance of maintaining self-control cannot be overstated. It is not always essential to make significant adjustments to one's eating habits to eat better by changing all of one's eating habits. Over time, even a few minor adjustments can have a significant impact, leading to a maintained weight reduction and an improvement in overall health.

CHAPTER 5

WHAT SHOULD BE DONE NEXT: KEEPING A HEALTHY BODY MASS INDEX

Calculating your overall health is difficult, but there is one straightforward approach that many people rely on your body mass index (BMI).

The abbreviation for "body mass index" is "BMI." It considers your age, height, and weight and then assigns you a score on a chart that ranges from underweight to highly obese based on those three factors. The optimal range for a healthy weight is somewhere around the middle.

The body mass index (BMI) is a valuable tool for determining whether or not your weight is usually healthy; however, it does have some drawbacks, such as the fact that it does not consider how your fat and muscle are distributed in your body.

BMI is determined using the formula weight (in kilograms) / height (in meters), which can be found here.2.

You may determine your own BMI by following these steps and entering your height in inches and weight in pounds into a calculator:

First, multiply your height by itself; then, divide your weight in pounds (lbs) by the number you received from the first step; and last, multiply your most recent result by 703.

The following is a list of important information on BMI:

A body mass index that falls between 18.5 and 24.9 is considered healthy. • Being underweight (a BMI of 18.5 or lower) or overweight/obese (a BMI of 25 or higher) might raise your risk for various health problems.

According to a consensus statement from multiple organizations, including the World Health Organization (WHO), the American Heart Association (AHA), and the Centers for Disease Control and Prevention (CDC), adults should aim to get at least moderate-intensity aerobic exercise each week, to improve overall health outcomes.

Regular exercise, such as aerobic exercise, for at least 150 minutes per week can help you maintain a healthy BMI and reduce the risk of chronic illness.

To improve overall health outcomes, adults should aim to get at least moderate aerobic exercises weekly.

If your body mass index (BMI) increases by one unit, your body fat percentage will increase by one unit. This is typically presented as a percentage of 0–25% or 25–30%. If your BMI falls between 18.5 and 25, it implies that you have a healthy, typical amount of body fat. Overweight is explained as having a body mass index (BMI) between 30 and 40, while obesity is having a BMI of 40 or above.

There is a correlation between higher BMI values and increased risks of acquiring the following health issues:

- Ailments of the cardiovascular system
- Hypertension, also known as high blood pressure
- Type 2 diabetes and insulin resistance syndrome can result in type 2 diabetes and hyperglycemia. A medical disease known as hyperglycemia is when a person's blood sugar levels remain abnormally high over an extended period.
- Sleep apnea and other sleep problems.

HOW TO GET YOUR BMI DOWN

There are a lot of techniques to decrease your BMI, albeit they may not be precisely what you want "to do" in one session. Below, we will discuss some of the treatment alternatives recommended by medical professionals as being among the most helpful.

1. **Cut down on the number of calories you consume each day**

This is the most fundamental method for bringing down the level of your BMI. If you have been attempting to lose weight for some time but haven't succeeded, you may already be doing this. You may help reduce your total body fat levels and, as a result, lower your BMI by following a diet with a calorie deficit or by intermittently fasting for short periods. As long as you remain consistent, even seemingly insignificant adjustments can significantly impact over time.

2. **Move your body.**

Exercise generally speeds up your metabolism, resulting in more calorie burning and weight reduction. Additionally, it lifts your mood, lowers your stress levels, and makes it easier to get a good night's sleep. However, walking for thirty minutes daily is an excellent habit that will enhance your health and does not require you to work out so hard that you are exhausted and sweating.

3. Improve your diet

Transition to a diet that consists of many more whole foods, fruits, and vegetables and a lot less processed and quick food. Whole plant-based meals provide fiber, vitamins, and minerals that help you feel fuller for longer and aid in weight loss. To develop muscle and reduce fat more quickly, you should increase your consumption of lean protein food sources such as beans (other than soy), lentils, quinoa, chickpeas, or tofu. Also, ensure you get sufficient vitamin D through exposure to sunshine or dietary sources such as fortified non-dairy alternatives such as cereals and juices.

4. Take in a lot more water

Dehydration is a risk factor for various health problems, including headaches and constipation. Consuming more water can facilitate weight loss, improve digestion, bring about an improvement in the purity of skin, and prevent the formation of kidney stones. Because drinking 8–10 glasses of water daily benefits your overall health, you should make it a daily habit. In addition to helping you feel full, drinking water at room temperature or cold will help you stay full for longer, which will, in the long run, help you avoid overeating.

5. Make sure you get adequate rest

Getting enough sleep is essential to maintaining a robust and healthy body. It also has a significant positive impact on your cognitive functioning, your mood, and your general stress levels. Because most of us eat more at night, not getting enough sleep might make it easier to lose weight and possibly contribute to obesity. Your cortisol levels will decrease due to sleep, which is beneficial given that elevated cortisol levels in the blood can lead to reduced sensitivity to insulin and long-term weight gain.

Always aim to obtain at least eight hours of sleep every night and maintain healthy sleeping habits. Put your mobile phone and other electronic devices away at least an hour before bedtime, wear comfortable clothes, and sleep in a cold and dark place.

ADVANTAGES TO ONE'S HEALTH OF MAINTAINING A HEALTHY BODY MASS INDEX

When it comes to maintaining a healthy body mass index, it's not enough to just be able to fit into a given size of clothing or reach a specific figure on the scale. Maintaining a healthy BMI is related to many positive health advantages. You can lower your chance of acquiring chronic sicknesses such as type 2 diabetes, cardiovascular disease, high blood pressure, and even some forms of cancer if you maintain a weight that is within the healthy range.

In addition, keeping a healthy body mass index (BMI) can assist in improving your energy levels, bolstering your immune system, and overall quality of life. It is important to remember that even minimal adjustments to one's lifestyle can, over time, significantly influence one's ability to maintain a healthy body mass index (BMI). Every step towards a healthy body mass index (BMI), whether through regular exercise, a balanced diet, or just adding more movement into your everyday routine, is a step towards a healthier life.

EFFECTS OF EXERCISE ON BMI

According to a declaration reached by a consensus of prominent health organizations, consistent aerobic activity that lasts for at least 150 minutes per week can lead to considerable decreases in body mass index. It is possible to enhance one's body composition by engaging in activities of moderate intensity, such as brisk walking, running, or cycling. This can be achieved by decreasing adipose mass and increasing lean muscle mass, which both contribute to a lower BMI score. However, it is essential to remember that the number and intensity of physical activity required for optimal BMI reduction may vary based on individual features such as age, sex, and overall health state. This is something that should be kept in mind at all times. It is usually suggested to consult with a healthcare practitioner before beginning a new fitness program.

PHYSICAL ACTIVITY THAT LEADS TO THE MOST SIGNIFICANT REDUCTIONS IN BMI

Consistency is the most critical factor when it comes to lowering your BMI through exercise. Combining several types of physical activity, including cardiovascular and strength training, is essential to get the most out of your workout program. Running, swimming, and cycling are excellent forms of cardiovascular exercise that help promote weight reduction and fat burning since they raise the heart rate and burn many calories. Building lean muscle mass through resistance training with weights or bodyweight workouts will assist, which in turn assists in boosting metabolism, allowing you to burn more calories even when you're not actively doing anything.

It has also been demonstrated to help improve body mass index (BMI) when a person's regular regimen incorporates high-intensity interval training (HIIT). This sort of workout consists of brief intervals of exercise performed at a high intensity, followed by periods of rest or activity performed at a lower level. Workouts incorporating high-intensity interval training (HIIT) are time-efficient but demand total effort during high-intensity intervals. This makes them hard, but they are also excellent for reducing body fat and improving cardiovascular health.

HOW TO KEEP UP A CONSISTENT PATTERN OF PHYSICAL ACTIVITY

Keeping a regular fitness program can be made easier by developing attainable objectives and keeping track of one's progress toward those goals. First, you should focus on creating manageable and reasonable objectives, such as exercising for one hour thrice weekly. Monitor your advancement and provide yourself with incentives for achieving your objective by utilizing a fitness tracker or a smartphone application.

Finding someone to hold you accountable or becoming a member of a fitness group are also excellent options for maintaining your motivation. If you have someone to talk to about the highs and lows of the journey alongside you, it may make the experience more fun and less intimidating. Alternatively, enrolling in a fitness class or joining a group that exercises together might provide additional motivation for social connection and support.

"Gamifying" your exercises by using apps or other technology to turn your workouts into a game is one more enjoyable method to stick to a fitness program. Many popular fitness applications provide challenges, awards, and friendly rivalry among friends, which may make working out feel more like a game than a duty. If you want to improve your health via more consistent physical exercise, including these tactics in your daily routine may help you stay on track to accomplish that goal!

OTHER ASPECTS THAT PLAY A ROLE IN DETERMINING BMI

It is, without a doubt, one of the most essential components in keeping a healthy BMI to engage in regular physical activity. Nevertheless, other, less evident aspects of your lifestyle can also affect both your weight and the makeup of your body. For example, research has shown that persistent worry and stress can lead to bad dietary choices and overeating, contributing to higher BMIs. Even if a person maintains the same amount of calories in their diet while taking some drugs, like antidepressants or birth control pills, the individual may experience weight gain as a side effect. Therefore, it is crucial to consider these external influences while monitoring the development of your BMI and making any required modifications to the routine you follow to maintain your general health.

The amount of physical activity a person does outside of their regular exercises is another key element influencing BMI. Even if you exercise consistently for an hour each day, sitting for lengthy periods during the day can still harm your metabolism and overall health outcomes over time. As a result, it is encouraged to strive for 10,000 steps per day or more by participating in light activities such as walking at lunch breaks or taking regular standing breaks during desk work hours whenever possible. These seemingly little adjustments, when added together, have a cumulative effect on lowering sedentary behavior and enhancing insulin sensitivity. This, in turn, leads to improved metabolic processes, which then leads to improved health outcomes, including the maintenance of healthy BMIs over the long run.

THE RELATIONSHIP BETWEEN DIET AND BMI

A well-balanced diet, which may be accomplished through adequate portion management, is required to keep a healthy body mass index (BMI). Consuming food in moderately sized increments throughout the day can assist in controlling calorie intake and preventing overeating. Adding to the amount of fruits and vegetables consumed during meals is one way to increase the amount of nutrient-dense and calorie-conscious foods consumed. When you eat less processed foods, you consume fewer items with added sugars, bad fats, and extra salt typically associated with these foods. Individuals can increase their body mass index and general health by implementing these dietary adjustments.

IMPROVING ONE'S BODY MASS INDEX (BMI) VIA BETTER MANAGEMENT OF SLEEP AND STRESS

Improving your body mass index (BMI) requires essential components, including stress

management and adequate sleep each night. A lack of sleep and unrestrained stress levels can lead to weight increase. Because it is crucial to prioritize these areas for general health development, it is important to note that both of these factors can contribute to weight gain. The practice of activities such as yoga or meditation can help regulate stress levels, but when dealing with chronic difficulties related to sleep or stress, it may be important to seek the assistance of a professional.

Make it a point to obtain at least seven hours of excellent sleep every night.

Experiment with different relaxing methods, such as deep breathing exercises, yoga, or meditation.

If you deal with ongoing problems connected to sleep or stress, you should seriously consider getting some professional assistance.

KEY POINT

When striving to maintain a healthy body mass index (BMI), many people have difficulty determining the appropriate quantity of physical activity. However, it is critical to remember that every person is unique and that the things that are successful for some people cannot be successful for others. Pay attention to what your body is telling you and discover an exercise level that you can maintain and find pleasurable over the long run.

In conclusion, while there are broad recommendations for the amount of weekly physical activity that we should strive for, the most important thing is to develop a routine tailored to your needs and preferences. Exercise of any kind, including low-impact activities like walking or yoga, is preferable to exercise of no kind at all. High-intensity exercises are beneficial, but so is a movement of any kind. We may better regulate our weight and keep a healthy body mass index if we include activity in our daily routines and pay attention to the requirements of our bodies.

CONCLUSION

People must continue their weight reduction regimen by taking particular actions to avoid missing out on the delicious treats they are used to eating while on the program. Regarding lowering the risk of being obese, the two most important things to remember are portion management and balanced diet choices. In addition, be sure to do regular exercise to cut down on the fat that has been collected.

You are the one who must take responsibility for maintaining a healthy lifestyle while indulging in some of your favorite indulgences. The purpose of the several stages that have been outlined here is to act as a guide.